The Definitive Comfort Food Guide for Tasty Meals

The best 50 tasty comfort food recipes for everyday meals

Orlando Bryant

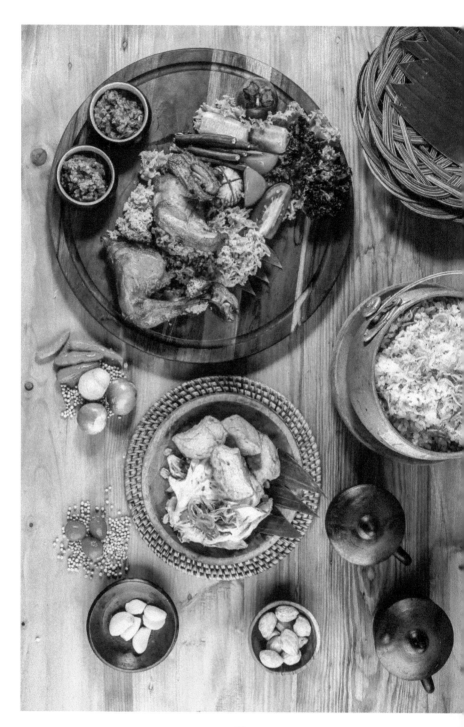

Table of Contents

Baked Apple

Preparation time: 5 minutes | Cooking Time: 20 minutes | Servings: 4

Ingredients:

¼ c. Water

¼ tsp. Nutmeg

¼ tsp. Cinnamon

1 ½ tsp. Melted ghee

2 tbsp. Raisins

2 tbsp. Chopped walnuts

1 medium apple

Directions:

Preparing the ingredients. Preheat your instant crisp air fryer to 350 degrees.

Slice the apple in half and discard some of the flesh from the center.

Place into the frying pan.

Mix remaining ingredients together except water.

Spoon mixture to the middle of apple halves.

Pour water overfilled apples.

Air frying. Place pan with apple halves into the instant crisp air fryer, close the air fryer lid.

Select bake, bake 20 minutes.

Nutrition:

Calories 199, Fat 9g, Protein 1g, Sugar 3g.

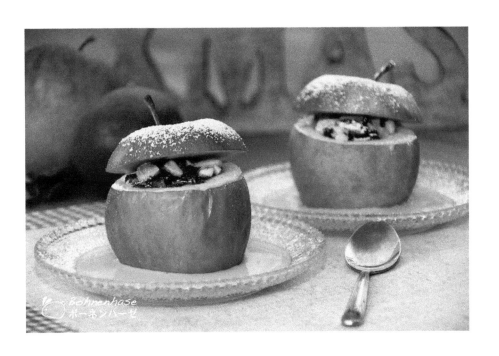

Coffee and Blueberry Cake

Preparation time: 5 minutes | Cooking Time: 35 minutes | Servings: 6

Ingredients:

1 cup white sugar

1 egg

1/2 cup butter, softened

1/2 cup fresh or frozen blueberries

1/2 cup sour cream

1/2 teaspoon baking powder

1/2 teaspoon ground cinnamon

1/2 teaspoon vanilla extract

1/4 cup brown sugar

1/4 cup chopped pecans

1/8 teaspoon salt

1-1/2 teaspoons confectioners' sugar for dusting

3/4 cup and 1 tablespoon all-purpose flour

Directions:

Preparing the ingredients. In a small bowl, whisk well pecans, cinnamon, and brown sugar.

In a blender, blend well all wet ingredients. Add dry ingredients except for confectioner's sugar and blueberries. Blend well until smooth and creamy.

Lightly grease the baking pan of the instant crisp air fryer with cooking spray.

Pour half of the batter into the pan. Sprinkle half of the pecan mixture on top. Pour the remaining batter. And then topped with the remaining pecan mixture.

Cover pan with foil.

Air frying. Close the air fryer lid. Select bake, and cook for 35 minutes, at 330°f.

Serve and enjoy with a dusting of confectioner's sugar.

Nutrition:

Calories 471, fat 24g, protein 4.1g, sugar 6g.

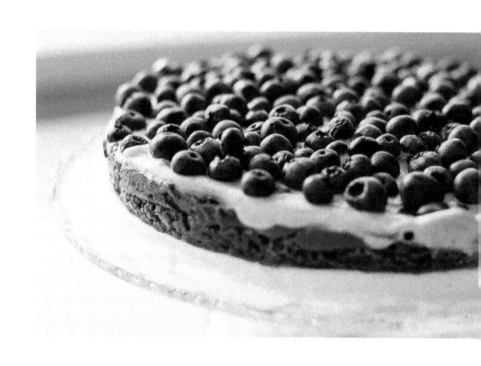

Roasted Chickpeas

Preparation time: 5 minutes | Cooking Time: 10 minutes | Servings: 2

Ingredients:

1 tbsp. Sweetener

1 tbsp. Cinnamon

1 c. Chickpeas

Directions:

Preparing the ingredients. Preheat an instant crisp air fryer to 390° F.

Rinse and drain chickpeas.

Mix all ingredients together and add to an instant crisp air fryer.

Air frying. Close the air fryer lid. Select bake, cook 10 minutes

Nutrition:

Calories 111, Fat 19g, Protein 16g, Sugar 5g.

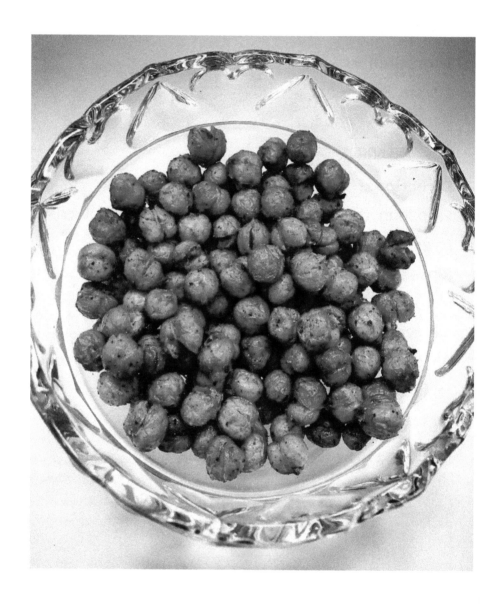

Cherry-Choco bars

Preparation time: 5 minutes | Cooking Time: 15 minutes | Servings: 8

Ingredients:

¼ teaspoon salt

½ cup almonds, sliced

½ cup chia seeds

½ cup dark chocolate, chopped

½ cup dried cherries, chopped

½ cup prunes, pureed

½ cup quinoa, cooked

¾ cup almond butter

1/3 cup honey

2 cups old-fashioned oats

2 tablespoon coconut oil

Directions:

Preparing the ingredients. Preheat the instant crisp air fryer to 375°f.

In a mixing bowl, combine the oats, quinoa, chia seeds, almond, cherries, and chocolate.

In a saucepan, heat the almond butter, honey, and coconut oil.

Pour the butter mixture over the dry mixture. Add salt and prunes.

Mix until well combined.

Pour over a baking dish that can fit inside the instant crisp air fryer.

Air frying. Close the air fryer lid. Select bake, cook for 15 minutes at 375°f.

Let it cool for an hour before slicing into bars.

Nutrition:

Calories 321, Fat 17g, Protein 7g, Sugar 5g.

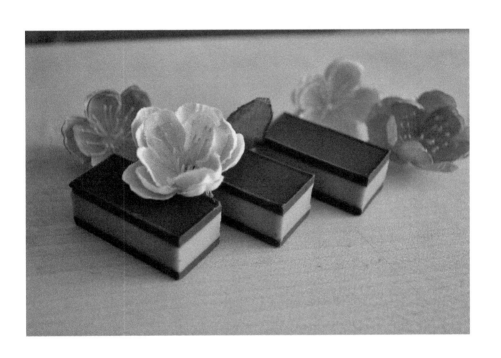

Cinnamon Fried Bananas

Preparation time: 5 minutes | Cooking Time: 10 minutes | Servings: 2-3

Ingredients:

1 c. Panko breadcrumbs

3 tbsp. Cinnamon

½ c. Almond flour

3 egg whites

8 ripe bananas

3 tbsp. Vegan coconut oil

Directions:

Preparing the ingredients. Heat coconut oil and add breadcrumbs.

Mix around 2-3 minutes until golden.

Pour into a bowl.

Peel and cut bananas in half.

Roll the half of each banana into flour, eggs, and crumb mixture.

Air frying. Place into the instant crisp air fryer.

Close the air fryer lid. Select bake and cook for 10 minutes at 280° F.

A great addition to a healthy banana split!

Nutrition:

Calories 219, Fat 10g, Protein 3g, Sugar 5g.

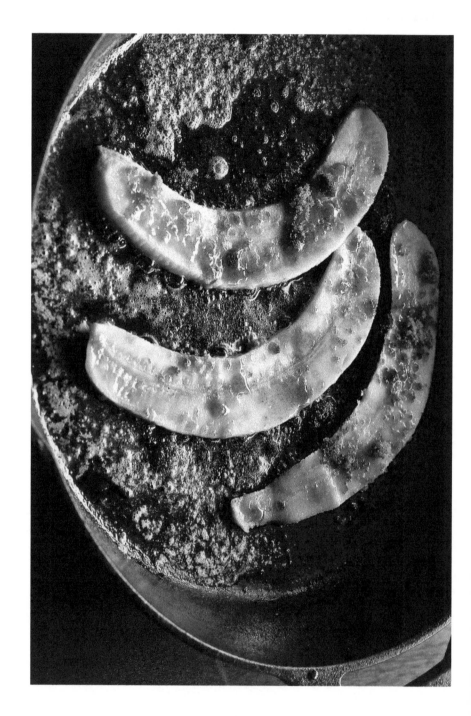

Buffalo Cauliflower Bites

Preparation Time: 10 minutes | Cooking Time: 14 minutes | Servings: 2

Ingredients:

3 cups cauliflower florets

2 eggs, lightly beaten

1/4 cup cornstarch

2 cups breadcrumbs

1 tsp onion powder

1 tsp garlic powder

1/2 cup hot sauce

Directions:

In a shallow bowl, mix breadcrumbs, cornstarch, onion powder, and garlic powder.

In a small bowl, add eggs.

Spray Pressure Pot multi-level air fryer basket with cooking spray.

Dip cauliflower florets in egg then coat with breadcrumb mixture and place into the air fryer basket and place basket into the Pressure Pot.

Seal pot with air fryer lid and select air fry mode then set the temperature to 380° F and timer for 12 minutes. Turn cauliflower florets halfway through.

Toss cauliflower florets into the hot sauce and serve.

Nutrition:

Calories 603, Fat 10.5g, Carbohydrates 103.6g, Sugar 12.1g, Protein 23.6g, Cholesterol 164mg.

Parmesan Brussels Sprouts

Preparation Time: 10 minutes | Cooking Time: 14 minutes | Servings: 4

Ingredients:

1 lb Brussel sprouts, cleaned and halved

2 tbsp olive oil

1/2 cup parmesan cheese, grated

Pepper

Salt

Directions:

Add Brussel sprouts, oil, cheese, pepper, and salt into the mixing bowl and toss well.

Spray Pressure Pot multi-level air fryer basket with cooking spray.

Add brussels sprouts into the air fryer basket and place basket into the Pressure Pot.

Seal pot with air fryer lid and select air fry mode then set the temperature to 350° F and timer for 14 minutes. Stir halfway through.

Serve and enjoy.

Nutrition:

Calories 145, Fat 9.8g, Carbohydrates 10.7g, Sugar 2.5g, Protein 7.5g, Cholesterol 8mg.

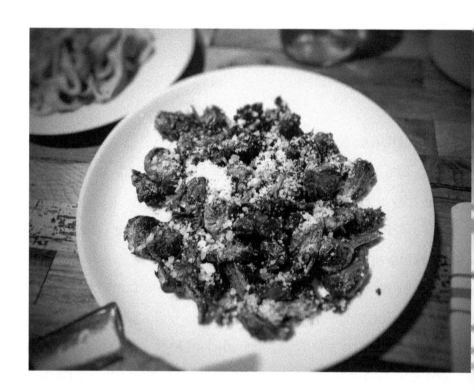

Bean, Tomato and Sour Cream Dip

Preparation time:30 minutes | Cooking Time: 10 minutes

Servings 12

Ingredients:

2 cups dried pinto beans, soaked overnight

2 14.5-ounce cans of tomatoes

1 teaspoon sweet paprika

1 teaspoon mustard powder

1 red chili pepper, minced

1 cup beef bone broth

1 teaspoon marjoram, dried

2 cloves garlic, minced

1/2 cup shallots, chopped

2 heaping tablespoons fresh chives, roughly chopped

1/4 teaspoon ground bay leaves

1 cup sour cream

Sea salt and ground black pepper, to taste

Directions:

Add the beans, garlic, shallots, chili pepper, tomatoes, broth, salt, black pepper, paprika, mustard powder, marjoram, and ground bay leaves to your Pressure Pot.

Secure the lid. Choose "Bean/Chili" mode and High pressure; cook for 25 minutes. Once cooking is complete, use a natural pressure release; carefully remove the lid.

Transfer the bean mixture to your food processor; mix until everything is creamy and smooth. Serve topped with sour cream and fresh chives. Enjoy!

Nutrition:

Calories 154, Fat 2.6g, Carbs 25.1g, Protein 8.3g, Sugars 3.1g.

Turnip and Sultana Dip with Pecans

Preparation Time: 10 minutes | Cooking Time: 15 Minutes | Servings: 4

Ingredients:

1 cup Water

2 pounds turnips, peeled and chopped

½ cup Sultanas

1 tbsp Vinegar

1 tbsp Olive Oil

¼ tsp Sea Salt

¼ tsp Black Pepper

Directions:

Heat oil on sauté at high, and cook turnips, until softened, for about 3 minutes. Stir in sultanas and water. Seal the lid, select the pressure cook/manual for 2 minutes at high pressure. Do a quick release.

Drain turnips and sultanas, and place in a food processor. Add some of the cooking water in, to make it creamier. Add vinegar, salt, and pepper, and pulse until smooth. Serve topped with chopped pecans.

Nutrition:

Calories 273, Carbs 45g, Fat 10g, Protein 5g.

Zestful Pea and Avocado Dip

Preparation Time: 25 minutes | Cooking Time: 15 Minutes | Servings: 4

Ingredients:

1 ½ cups dried Green Peas

1 tbsp Lime Juice

1 Avocado, peeled and deseeded

¼ tsp Pepper

1 Garlic Clove, peeled

2 cups Water

Directions:

Combine the water and peas in the pressure cooker. Seal the lid and turn clockwise to seal. Select the pressure cook/manual mode, set the timer to 16 minutes at high pressure. When the timer goes off, release the pressure quickly. Drain the peas and transfer them to a food processor. Add the remaining Ingredients, and pulse until smooth and creamy.

Nutrition:

Calories 123, Carbs 15g, Fat 8g, Protein 5g.

Beef Olive Balls

Preparation Time: 10 minutes | Cooking Time: 14 minutes | Servings: 4

Ingredients:

1 lb ground beef

1 tbsp oregano, chopped

1 tbsp breadcrumbs

1 tbsp chives, chopped

1 cup olives, pitted and chopped

Pepper

Salt

Directions:

Add all ingredients into the mixing bowl and mix until well combined.

Place the dehydrating tray in a multi-level air fryer basket and place basket in the Pressure Pot.

Make small balls from the meat mixture and place them on a dehydrating tray.

Seal pot with air fryer lid and select air fry mode then set the temperature to 400° F and timer for 14 minutes.

Turn meatballs halfway through.

Serve and enjoy.

Nutrition:

Calories 260, Fat 10.9g, Carbohydrates 4.1g, Sugar 0.2g, Protein 35.1g, Cholesterol 101mg.

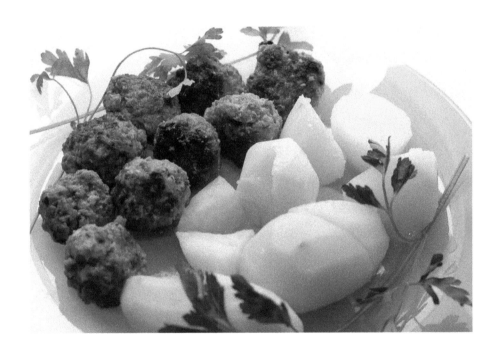

Moist Chocolate Cake

Preparation Time: 10 minutes | Cooking Time: 25 minutes | Servings: 8

Ingredients:

1 egg

1 tsp baking soda

1 tsp baking powder

3 tbsp cocoa powder

1 cup of sugar

1 cup all-purpose flour

1 tsp vanilla

1/4 cup butter

1 cup boiling water

1/4 tsp salt

Directions:

Spray a baking dish with cooking spray and set it aside.

Add butter and boiling water in a mixing bowl and beat until butter is melted.

Add vanilla and egg and beat until well combined.

In a medium bowl, mix flour, baking soda, baking powder, cocoa powder, sugar, and salt.

Add egg mixture into the flour mixture and beat until well combined.

Pour batter into prepared baking dish.

Place steam rack in the Pressure Pot then places a baking dish on top of the rack.

Seal pot with air fryer lid and select bake mode then set the temperature to 350° F and timer for 25 minutes.

Serve and enjoy.

Nutrition:

Calories 216, Fat 6.7g, Carbohydrates 38.5g, Sugar 25.2g, Protein 2.7g, Cholesterol 36mg.

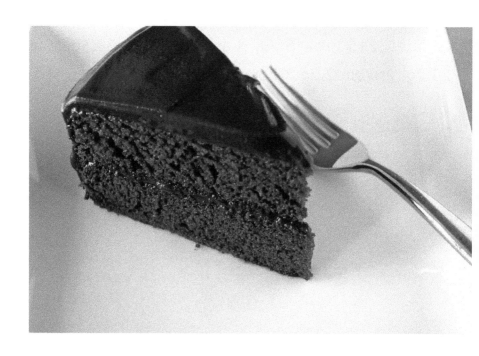

Key Lime Pie

Preparation Time: 10 minutes | Cooking Time: 30 minutes | Servings: 1

Ingredients For the filling:

2 eggs

1/4 cup condensed milk

2 tbsp fresh lime juice

For crust:

1 tbsp butter, melted

1/4 cup crushed cracker crumbs

Directions:

Mix crushed cracker crumbs and melted butter.

Add crushed cracker mixture into the ramekin and press down with the back of the spoon.

Place the dehydrating tray in a multi-level air fryer basket and place basket in the Pressure Pot.

Place ramekin on a dehydrating tray.

Seal pot with air fryer lid and select bake mode then set the temperature to 350° F and timer for 15 minutes.

Once done then remove the ramekin from the pot and set it aside to cool.

For filling: In a small bowl, whisk eggs with condensed milk and lime juice until smooth.

Pour egg mixture into baked crust.

Again, place the ramekin on a dehydrating tray.

Seal pot with air fryer lid and select bake mode then set the temperature to 350° F and timer for 15 minutes.

Serve and enjoy.

Nutrition:

Calories 589, Fat 29g, Carbohydrates 67g, Sugar 47.8g, Protein 18.9g, Cholesterol 384mg.

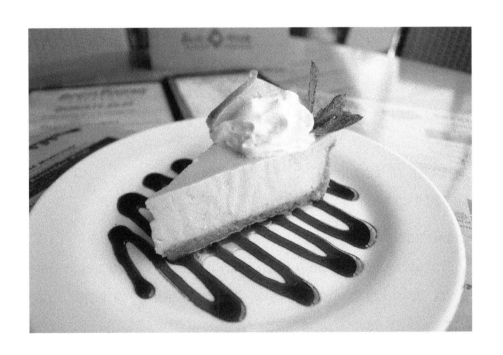

Choco Chip Brownies

Preparation Time: 10 minutes | Cooking Time: 25 minutes | Servings: 8

Ingredients:

2 eggs

1/2 cup olive oil

1 tsp vanilla

1/2 cup chocolate chips

1/4 tsp baking powder

1/3 cup cocoa powder

1/2 cup flour

1 cup of sugar

1/2 tsp salt

Directions:

Spray a baking dish with cooking spray and set it aside.

In a mixing bowl, mix flour, baking powder, cocoa powder, sugar, and salt.

Add eggs, oil, and vanilla and stir until combined.

Add chocolate chips and stir well.

Pour batter into the baking dish.

Place steam rack in the Pressure Pot then places baking dish on top of the rack.

Seal pot with air fryer lid and select bake mode then set the temperature to 350° F and timer for 25 minutes. Serve and enjoy.

Nutrition:

Calories 312, Fat 17.4g, Carbohydrates 39.4g, Sugar 30.6g, Protein 3.6g, Cholesterol 43mg.

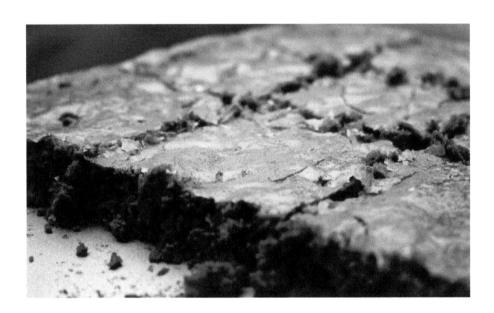

Moist Nutella Brownies

Preparation Time: 10 minutes | Cooking Time: 20 minutes | Servings: 8

Ingredients:

2 eggs

1/2 cup all-purpose flour

1 1/4 cup Nutella chocolate hazelnut spread

1 tsp kosher salt

Directions:

Spray a baking dish with cooking spray and set it aside.

In a mixing bowl, mix eggs, Nutella, flour, and salt until well combined.

Pour batter into the prepared baking dish.

Place steam rack in the Pressure Pot then places baking dish on top of the rack.

Seal pot with air fryer lid and select bake mode then set the temperature to 350° F and timer for 20 minutes.

Serve and enjoy.

Nutrition:

Calories 294, Fat 16.2g, Carbohydrates 32.3g, Sugar 26.4g, Protein 4.7g, Cholesterol 41mg.

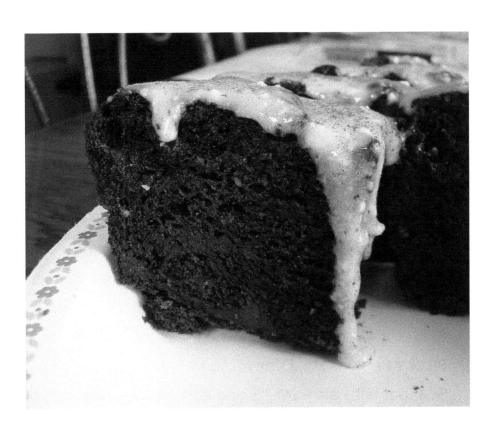

Lemon Mousse

Preparation Time: 10 minutes | Cooking Time: 12 minutes | Servings: 2

Ingredients:

2 oz cream cheese, soft

1/2 tsp liquid stevia

2 tbsp fresh lemon juice

1/2 cup heavy cream

Pinch of salt

Directions:

Spray 2 ramekins with cooking spray and set aside.

In a bowl, beat together cream cheese, sweetener, lemon juice, heavy cream, and salt until smooth.

Pour cream cheese mixture into the prepared ramekins.

Place the dehydrating tray in a multi-level air fryer basket and place basket in the Pressure Pot.

Place ramekins on a dehydrating tray.

Seal pot with air fryer lid and select bake mode then set the temperature to 350° F and timer for 12 minutes.

Serve and enjoy.

Nutrition:

Calories 206, Fat 21.1g, Carbohydrates 1.9g, Sugar 0.4g, Protein 2.9g, Cholesterol 72mg.

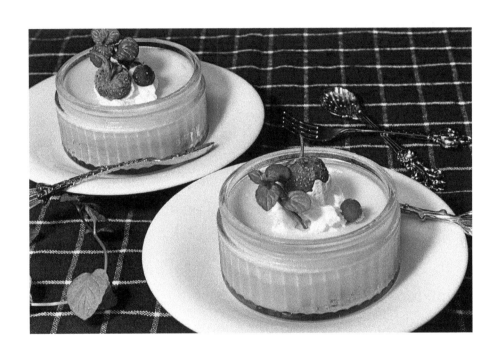

Healthy Almond Cookies

Preparation Time: 10 minutes | Cooking Time: 30 minutes | Servings: 12

Ingredients:

1/2 cup almonds, chopped

1 1/2 cups almond meal

1 tsp baking powder

1/2 tsp vanilla

1 cup of coconut sugar

1/4 cup coconut oil, melted

1 tbsp ground flaxseed

Directions:

In a small bowl, mix ground flaxseed and 2 tbsp water and set aside.

In a mixing bowl, whisk oil, vanilla, sugar, and flaxseed mixture until well combined.

Add almond meal, almonds, and baking powder and mix until well combined.

Place the dehydrating tray in a multi-level air fryer basket and place basket in the Pressure Pot.

Line dehydrating tray with parchment paper.

Make cookies from the mixture and place some cookies on the dehydrating tray.

Seal pot with air fryer lid and select air fry mode then set the temperature to 340 ° F and timer for 30 minutes.

Bake remaining cookies using the same method.

Serve and enjoy.

Nutrition:

Calories 95, Fat 8.6g, Carbohydrates 3.5g, Sugar 0.3g, Protein 1.9g, Cholesterol 0mg.

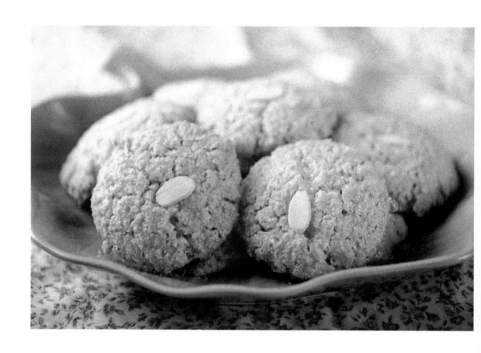

Vanilla Brownie

Preparation Time: 10 minutes | Cooking Time: 20 minutes | Servings: 4

Ingredients:

1 egg

1/4 cup cocoa powder

1 tsp vanilla

2 tbsp olive oil

1/3 cup flour

2 tbsp sugar

1/4 cup chocolate chips

Directions:

Spray a baking dish with cooking spray and set it aside.

In a bowl, whisk egg, vanilla, oil, and sugar.

In a mixing bowl, mix flour and cocoa powder.

Add egg mixture into the flour mixture and mix until well combined.

Pour batter into the prepared baking dish.

Place steam rack in the Pressure Pot then places baking dish on top of the rack.

Seal pot with air fryer lid and select bake mode then set the temperature to 320° F and timer for 20 minutes.

Serve and enjoy.

Nutrition:

Calories 207, Fat 12g, Carbohydrates 23.4g, Sugar 11.7g, Protein 4.2g, Cholesterol 43mg.

Lava Cakes

Preparation Time: 10 minutes | Cooking Time: 10 minutes | Servings: 4

Ingredients:

2 eggs

3.5 oz dark chocolate, melted

1 1/2 tbsp self-rising flour

3 tbsp sugar

3.5 oz butter, melted

Directions:

Spray four ramekins with cooking spray and set them aside.

In a bowl, beat eggs and sugar until frothy.

Add melted chocolate, flour, and butter and fold well.

Pour batter into the prepared ramekins.

Place the dehydrating tray in a multi-level air fryer basket and place basket in the Pressure Pot.

Place ramekins on a dehydrating tray.

Seal pot with air fryer lid and select air fry mode then set the temperature to 375° F and timer for 10 minutes.

Serve and enjoy.

Nutrition:

Calories 387, Fat 29.7g, Carbohydrates 26.2g, Sugar 22g, Protein 5.2g, Cholesterol 141mg.

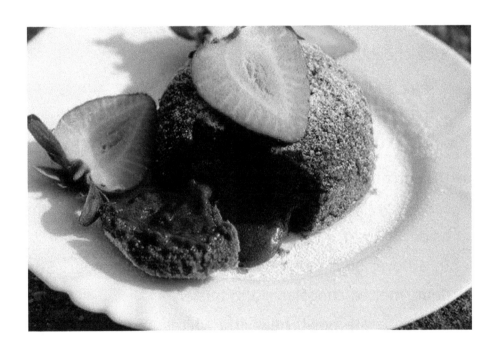

Chocolate Souffle

Preparation Time: 10 minutes | Cooking Time: 15 minutes | Servings: 2

Ingredients:

2 egg whites

2 egg yolks

1/2 tsp vanilla

3 oz chocolate, melted

3 tbsp sugar

2 tbsp flour

1/4 cup butter, melted

Directions:

Spray two ramekins with cooking spray and set them aside.

In a bowl, beat egg yolks with vanilla and sugar. Stir in flour, melted chocolate, and butter.

In a separate bowl, beat egg whites and until stiff peak forms.

Slowly fold the egg white mixture into the egg yolk mixture.

Pour batter into the prepared ramekins.

Place the dehydrating tray in a multi-level air fryer basket and place basket in the Pressure Pot.

Place ramekins on a dehydrating tray.

Seal pot with air fryer lid and select bake mode then set the temperature to 330° F and timer for 15 minutes.

Serve and enjoy.

Nutrition:

Calories 601, Fat 40.3g, Carbohydrates 50.2g, Sugar 40.4g, Protein 10.6g, Cholesterol 281mg.

Squash and Cranberry Sauce

Preparation time: 10 minutes | Cooking Time: 7 minutes | Servings: 4

Ingredients:

¼ cup raisins

2 acorn squash, peeled and roughly chopped

14 ounces cranberry sauce, unsweetened

¼ teaspoon ground cinnamon

A pinch of sea salt and black pepper

Directions:

In your Pressure Pot, mix squash with cranberry sauce, raisins, cinnamon, salt, and pepper. Stir, cover, cook on High pressure for 7 minutes, divide into bowls and serve.

Enjoy!

Nutrition:

Calories 140, fat 3g, fiber 2g, carbs 3g, protein 4g.

Beef and Cabbage Hash

Preparation time: 10 minutes | Cooking Time: 16 minutes | Servings: 2

Ingredients:

1 tablespoon olive oil

1 yellow onion, chopped

2 cups cubed corned beef

2 garlic cloves, minced

½ cup beef stock

A pinch of salt and black pepper

1 pound cabbage, chopped

Directions:

Set your Pressure Pot to sauté mode, add oil and heat.

Add onion, stir and cook for 2 minutes.

Add garlic and cabbage, stir and sauté for 4 minutes more.

Add beef, stock, salt, and pepper. Stir, cover, and cook on High pressure for 10 minutes.

Divide into bowls and serve for breakfast.

Enjoy!

Nutrition:

Calories 160, fat 3g, fiber 3g, carbs 5g, protein 4g.

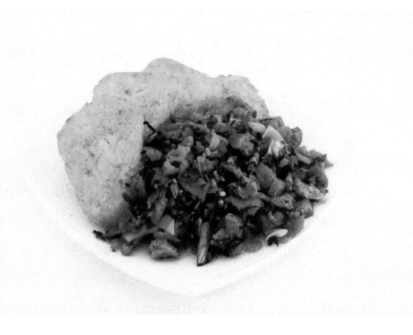

Chicken, Bacon and Veggie Omelet

Preparation time: 10 minutes | Cooking Time: 10 minutes | Servings: 1

Ingredients:

1-ounce rotisserie chicken, shredded

1 teaspoon mustard

1 tablespoon homemade keto mayonnaise

1 tomato, chopped

2 bacon slices, cooked and crumbled

3 eggs, whisked

1 small avocado, pitted, peeled, and chopped

Salt and black pepper to the taste

A drizzle of olive oil

Directions:

In a bowl, whisk eggs with chicken, mustard, mayo, tomato, bacon, avocado, salt, and pepper.

Set your Pressure Pot to sauté mode, add the oil, and heat. Add eggs mix, spread, and cook for 2 minutes.

Cover your Pressure Pot, cook your omelet on High pressure for 2 minutes, divide it between plates, and serve for breakfast.

Enjoy!

Nutrition:

Calories 237, fat 4g, fiber 6g, carbs 8g, protein 70g.

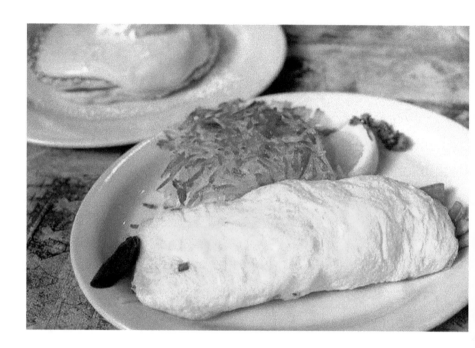

Nuts, Squash, and Apples Breakfast

Preparation time: 10 minutes | Cooking Time: 10 minutes | Servings: 4

Ingredients:

½ cup almonds, soaked for 12 hours, and drained

½ cup walnuts, soaked for 12 hours, and drained

2 apples, peeled, cored, and cubed

1 butternut squash, peeled and cubed

1 teaspoon ground cinnamon

1 tablespoon stevia

½ teaspoon ground nutmeg

1 cup coconut milk, unsweetened

Directions:

Put the almonds in your blender, pulse well, and transfer to your Pressure Pot.

Add walnuts, apples, squash, cinnamon, stevia, milk, and nutmeg. Stir, cover, and cook on High pressure for 10 minutes.

Divide into bowls and serve for breakfast.

Enjoy!

Nutrition:

Calories 140, fat 1g, fiber 2g, carbs 6g, protein 3g.

Shallot, Kale and Beef Breakfast

Preparation time: 10 minutes | Cooking Time: 10 minutes | Servings: 4

Ingredients:

1 1/3 cups shallots, chopped

1 cup kale, chopped

½ cup of water

2 tablespoons olive oil

2 teaspoons garlic, minced

8 eggs

2/3 cup celeriac, peeled and grated

1½ cups beef sausage, casings removed and chopped

Directions:

Set your Pressure Pot to Sauté mode, add the oil and heat. Add shallots, stir and sauté for 1 minute.

Add the celeriac, kale, water, and garlic, stir and sauté for 1 minute more.

Add beef sausage and eggs, stir, cover, and cook on High pressure for 6 minutes.

Divide this mix on plates and serve for breakfast.

Enjoy!

Nutrition:

Calories 150, fat 2g, fiber 2g, carbs 5g, protein 6g.

Strawberry and Coconut Breakfast

Preparation time: 10 minutes | Cooking Time: 10 minutes | Servings: 2

Ingredients:

3 tablespoons coconut flakes, unsweetened

2 tablespoon strawberries, chopped

1 cup of water

2/3 cup coconut milk, unsweetened

½ teaspoon stevia

Directions:

In your Pressure Pot, mix strawberries with coconut flakes, water, milk, and stevia. Stir, cover, and cook on High pressure for 10 minutes.

Divide into 2 bowls and serve for breakfast.

Enjoy!

Nutrition:

Calories 110, fat 12g, fiber 3g, carbs 3g, protein 3g.

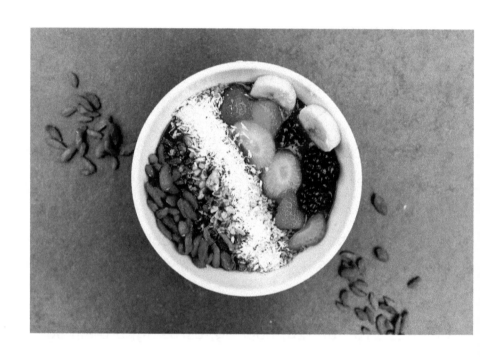

Chorizo and Veggies Mix

Preparation time: 10 minutes | Cooking Time: 15 minutes | Servings: 2

Ingredients:

1 pound chorizo, chopped

1 small yellow onion, chopped

2 garlic cloves, minced

4 bacon slices, chopped

½ cup beef stock

2 poblano peppers, chopped

1 cup chopped kale

8 mushrooms, chopped

½ cup chopped cilantro

1 avocado, peeled, pitted, and chopped

4 eggs

Directions:

Set your Pressure Pot to sauté mode, add chorizo and bacon. Stir and cook for 2 minutes.

Add garlic, onion, and poblano peppers, stir and cook for 2 minutes more.

Add kale, mushrooms, and stock, stir, make 4 holes in this mix and crack an egg into each hole. Cover pot and cook on High pressure for 4 minutes.

Divide this between plates, add avocado and cilantro on top and serve for breakfast.

Enjoy!

Nutrition:

Calories 160, fat 5g, fiber 3g, carbs 5g, protein 7g.

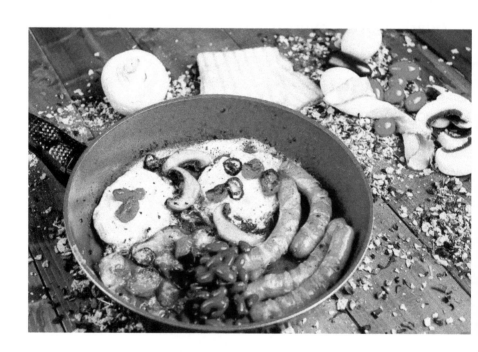

Vanilla and Espresso Coconut Oatmeal

Preparation time: 10 minutes | Cooking Time: 10 minutes | Servings: 4

Ingredients:

1 cup of coconut milk

1 cup coconut flakes

2 cups of water

2 tablespoons stevia

1 teaspoon espresso powder

2 teaspoons vanilla extract

Grated dark and bitter chocolate for serving

Directions:

In your Pressure Pot, mix coconut flakes with water, stevia, milk, and espresso powder. Stir, cover, and cook on High pressure for 10 minutes.

Add vanilla extract, stir, divide into bowls and serve with grated chocolate on top.

Enjoy!

Nutrition:

Calories 172, fat 2g, fiber 4g, carbs 7g, protein 8g.

Coconut and Pomegranate Oatmeal

Preparation time: 5 minutes | Cooking Time: 2 minutes | Servings: 2

Ingredients:

1 cup coconut, shredded, unsweetened

1 cup of water

¾ cup pomegranate juice

Seeds from 1 pomegranate

Directions:

In your Pressure Pot, mix coconut with water and pomegranate juice. Stir, cover, and cook on High pressure for 2 minutes.

Add pomegranate seeds, stir oatmeal, divide into bowls and serve for breakfast.

Enjoy!

Nutrition:

Calories 183, fat 3g, fiber 6g, carbs 9g, protein 6g.

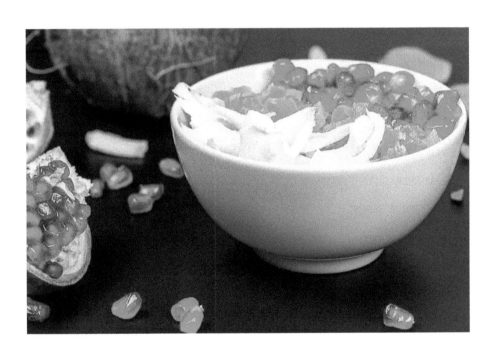

Cauliflower Rice Bowl

Preparation time: 5 minutes | Cooking Time: 7 minutes | Servings: 4

Ingredients:

1 cup rice cauliflower

½ cup coconut chips, unsweetened

1 cup coconut milk, unsweetened

3 tablespoons stevia

¼ cup raisins

¼ cup chopped almonds

A pinch of ground cinnamon

Directions:

In your Pressure Pot, mix cauliflower rice with coconut, coconut milk, stevia, raisins, almonds, and cinnamon. Stir, cover, and cook on High pressure for 7 minutes. Divide into bowls and serve for breakfast.

Enjoy!

Nutrition:

Calories 172, fat 8g, fiber 3g, carbs 7g, protein 10g.

Tomato and Zucchini Salad

Preparation time: 10 minutes | Cooking Time: 10 minutes | Servings: 4

Ingredients:

2 spring onions, chopped

1 pound cherry tomatoes, roughly cubed

2 zucchinis, sliced

1 tablespoon olive oil

2 garlic cloves, minced

1 tablespoon rosemary, chopped

1 tablespoon basil, chopped

½ cup tomato passata

1 tablespoon chives, chopped

A pinch of sea salt and black pepper

Directions:

Set your Pressure Pot on sauté mode add the oil, heat it, add the spring onions and the garlic, and sauté for 2-3 minutes.

Add tomatoes, zucchinis, and the rest of the ingredients except the chives, put the lid on, and cook on High for 8 minutes.

Release the pressure naturally for 10 minutes, divide the mix into bowls and serve for breakfast with the chives sprinkled on top.

Nutrition:

Calories 86, fat 4.1g, fiber 3.6g, carbs 5.8g, protein 3g.

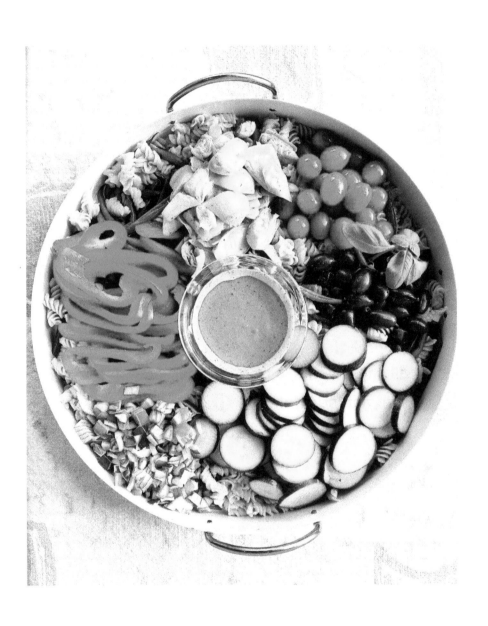

Creamy Apple Rhubarb Pudding

Preparation Time: 10 minutes | Cooking Time: 15 minutes | Servings: 6

Ingredients:

1 cup Arborio rice

2 rhubarb stalks, chopped

1/2 apple, peeled and chopped

1/2 cup water

1 cinnamon stick

1 tsp vanilla

1 1/2 cup milk

1 tsp cinnamon

Directions:

Add all ingredients into the inner pot of Pressure Pot duo crisp and stir well.

Seal the pot with a pressure-cooking lid and cook on high for 15 minutes.

Once done, release pressure using a quick release. Remove lid.

Stir well and serve.

Nutrition:

Calories 161, Fat 1.5g, Carbs 31.9g, Sugar 5g, Protein 4.3g, Cholesterol 5mg.

Blueberry Muffins

Preparation Time: 10 minutes | Cooking Time: 15 minutes | Servings: 4

Ingredients:

1 egg

3/4 cup blueberries

1/2 tsp vanilla

2 tbsp erythritol

1 tsp baking powder

2/3 cup almond flour

3 tbsp butter, melted

1/3 cup almond milk

Directions:

Add all ingredients into the large bowl and mix until combined.

Pour batter into the silicone muffin molds.

Place in Pressure Pot air fryer basket and place basket in the pot.

Seal the pot with an air fryer lid and select bake mode and cook at 320° F for 15 minutes.

Serve and enjoy.

Nutrition:

Calories 268, Fat 23.5g, Carbohydrates 17.3g, Sugar 11g, Protein 6.1g, Cholesterol 64mg.

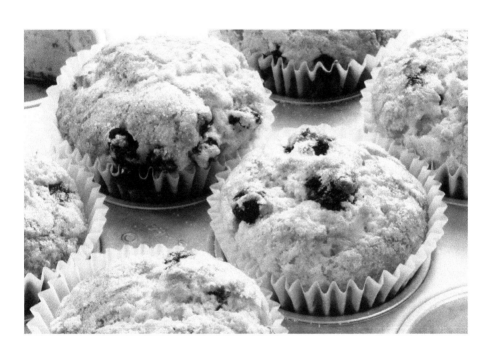

Vanilla Pumpkin Pudding

Preparation Time: 10 minutes | Cooking Time: 20 minutes | Servings: 6

Ingredients:

2 eggs

1/2 cup almond milk

1/2 tsp vanilla

1/2 tsp pumpkin pie spice

14 oz pumpkin puree

1/4 cup sugar

Directions:

Grease a 6-inch baking dish with cooking spray and set aside.

In a large bowl, whisk eggs with the remaining ingredients.

Pour mixture into the prepared dish and cover with foil.

Pour 1 1/2 cups of water into the inner pot of Pressure Pot duo crisp then place a steamer rack in the pot.

Place dish on top of the steamer rack.

Seal the pot with a pressure-cooking lid and cook on high for 20 minutes.

Once done, allow to release pressure naturally for 10 minutes then release remaining pressure using a quick release. Remove lid.

Carefully remove the dish from the pot and let it cool completely then place in the refrigerator for 5 hours before serving.

Serve and enjoy.

Nutrition:

Calories 122, Fat 6.4g, Carbohydrates 15g, Sugar 11.3g, Protein 3.1g, Cholesterol 55mg.

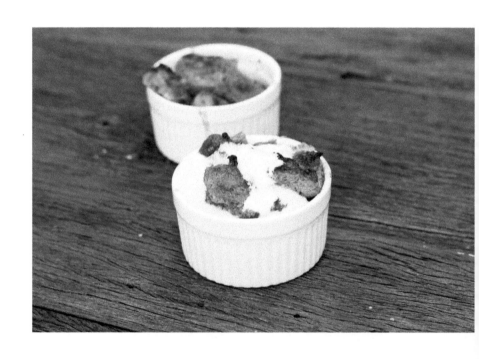

Cinnamon Bread Pudding

Preparation Time: 10 minutes | Cooking Time: 15 minutes | Servings: 2

Ingredients:

3 eggs, beaten

4 cups bread cube

3 tbsp raisins

1 cup almond milk

1/2 tsp cinnamon

1/2 tsp vanilla

1 tsp olive oil

Pinch of salt

Directions:

Place bread cubes in the oven-safe casserole dish.

In a bowl, mix remaining ingredients and pour over bread cubes. Cover dish with foil.

Pour 2 cups of water into the inner pot of Pressure Pot duo crisp then place steamer rack in the pot.

Place casserole dish on top of the steamer rack.

Seal the pot with a pressure-cooking lid and cook on high for 15 minutes.

Once done, allow to release pressure naturally for 10 minutes then release remaining pressure using a quick release. Remove lid.

Serve and enjoy.

Nutrition:

Calories 635, Fat 37.6g, Carbohydrates 58.5g, Sugar 12.7g, Protein 11.5g, Cholesterol 246mg.

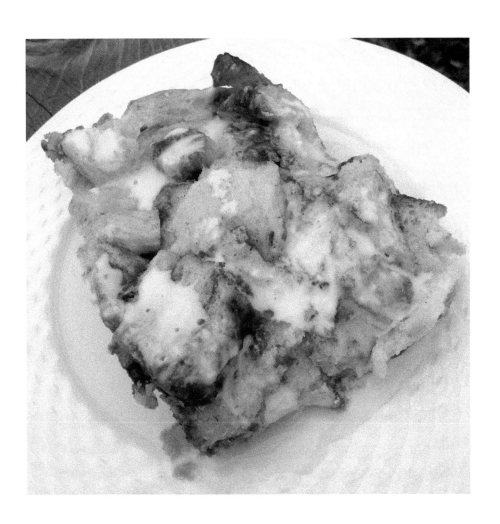

Cranberry Coconut Pudding

Preparation Time: 10 minutes | Cooking Time: 20 minutes | Servings: 6

Ingredients:

1 cup brown rice, rinsed and drained

1/2 cup coconut milk

1 1/2 cups milk

1 cup cranberries

1/4 cup sugar

1/2 tsp cinnamon

1/2 cup water

Directions:

Add all ingredients into the inner pot Pressure Pot duo crisp and stir well.

Seal the pot with a pressure-cooking lid and cook on high for 20 minutes.

Once done, allow to release pressure naturally. Remove lid.

Stir and serve.

Nutrition:

Calories 233, Fat 6.9g, Carbohydrates 38.4g, Sugar 12.4g, Protein 4.9g, Cholesterol 5mg.

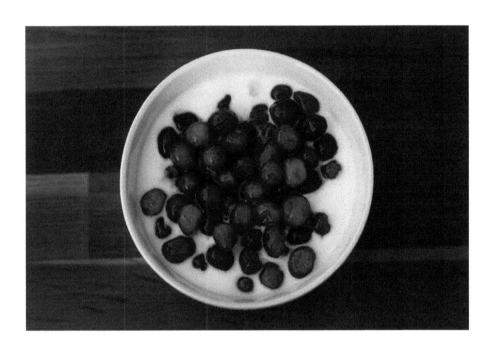

Vermicelli Pudding

Preparation Time: 10 minutes | Cooking Time: 3 minutes | Servings: 6

Ingredients:

1/3 cup vermicelli, roasted

2 tbsp ghee

1/4 cup cashews, slice

1/4 cup shredded coconut

1/4 cup raisins

1/4 cup almonds

1/4 cup sugar

5 cups of milk

Directions:

Add ghee into the inner pot of Pressure Pot duo crisp and set pot on sauté mode.

Add cashews and almonds and sauté for a minute.

Add raisins, coconut, and vermicelli, 3 cups milk, and sugar. Stir well.

Seal the pot with a pressure-cooking lid and cook on high for 2 minutes.

Once done, allow to release pressure naturally. Remove lid.

Add remaining milk and stir well.

Serve and enjoy.

Nutrition:

Calories 268, Fat 14.3g, Carbohydrates 28.7g, Sugar 21.9g, Protein 9.1g, Cholesterol 28mg.

Raspberry Cake

Preparation Time: 10 minutes | Cooking Time: 10 minutes | Servings: 8

Ingredients:

1/2 cup raspberries

5 egg yolks

1/4 cup heavy cream

1/2 cup coconut flour

1 tsp baking powder

3 tsp liquid stevia

1/4 cup butter

1/4 cup coconut oil

1/2 tsp vanilla

Directions:

Add all dry ingredients except raspberries in a large bowl and mix well.

Add all wet ingredients and beat using a blender until well combined.

Spray 6-inch spring-form baking dish with cooking spray.

Pour batter into the prepared baking dish and top with raspberries.

Pour 2 cups of water into the inner pot of Pressure Pot duo crisp then place steamer rack in the pot.

Place baking dish on top of the steamer rack.

Seal the pot with a pressure-cooking lid and cook on high for 10 minutes.

Once done, release pressure using a quick release. Remove lid.

Serve and enjoy.

Nutrition:

Calories 192, Fat 17.6g, Carbohydrates 6.7g, Sugar 0.4g, Protein 2.9g, Cholesterol 152mg.

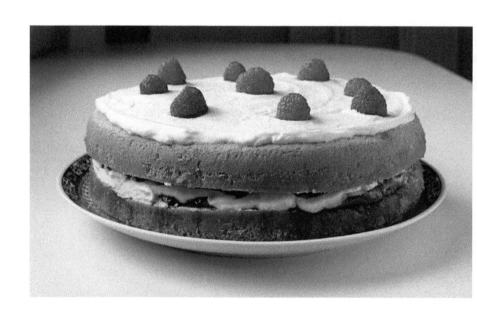

Chocolate Rice Pudding

Preparation Time: 10 minutes | Cooking Time: 15 minutes | Servings: 6

Ingredients:

2 eggs, beaten

1 cup rice, rinsed

2 tbsp cocoa powder

1/2 tsp vanilla

5 cups of coconut milk

1 tbsp coconut oil

1/2 cup sugar

Directions:

Add all ingredients into the inner pot of Pressure Pot duo crisp and set pot on sauté mode. Stir constantly and bring to boil.

Seal the pot with a pressure-cooking lid and cook on high for 15 minutes.

Once done, allow to release pressure naturally. Remove lid.

Stir well and serve.

Nutrition:

Calories 681, Fat 51.9g, Carbohydrates 53.5g, Sugar 23.6g, Protein 9g, Cholesterol 55mg.

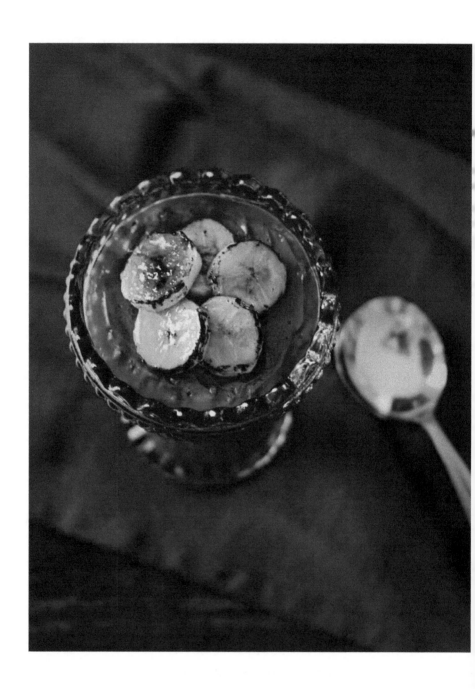

Choco Fudge

Preparation Time: 10 minutes | Cooking Time: 15 minutes | Servings: 8

Ingredients:

5 eggs

1/2 cup cocoa powder

1/2 cup dark chocolate, chopped

2 cups almond flour

1 tsp baking soda

1/2 tsp vanilla

2 tbsp erythritol

3/4 tsp baking powder

1/2 cup almond milk

Pinch of salt

Directions:

Add all dry ingredients into the large bowl and mix to combine.

Add remaining ingredients and beat using a blender until well combined.

Pour 2 cups of water into the inner pot of Pressure Pot duo crisp then place steamer rack in the pot.

Pour batter in the oven-safe baking dish and place on top of the steamer rack.

Seal the pot with a pressure-cooking lid and cook on high for 15 minutes.

Once done, release pressure using a quick release. Remove lid.

Serve and enjoy.

Nutrition:

Calories 311, Fat 23.4g, Carbohydrates 17.7g, Sugar 7.5g, Protein 11.6g, Cholesterol 105mg.

Delicious Lime Pudding

Preparation Time: 10 minutes | Cooking Time: 3 minutes | Servings: 4

Ingredients:

1/4 cup coconut milk

3/4 tsp lime zest, grated

1/2 tsp orange extract

1 tbsp swerve

1/4 cup heavy whipping cream

1/4 cup coconut cream

1 tsp agar powder

1 tbsp coconut oil

Directions:

Add coconut oil into the inner pot of Pressure Pot duo crisp and set the pot on sauté mode.

Add coconut milk, whipping cream, and coconut cream to the pot and stir constantly.

Add orange extract, swerve, and agar powder. Stir constantly and cook for 2-3 minutes.

Turn off the pot and pour the potting mix into the ramekins.

Sprinkle lime zest on top of each ramekin.

Place ramekins in the fridge for 1-2 hours.

Serve and enjoy.

Nutrition:

Calories 159, Fat 12.8g, Carbohydrates 11.6g, Sugar 10.1g, Protein 0.7g, Cholesterol 10mg.

Thai Coconut Rice

Preparation Time: 10 minutes | Cooking Time: 8 minutes | Servings: 4

Ingredients:

1 cup Thai sweet rice

14 oz coconut milk

1 1/2 cups water

1/2 tsp cornstarch

4 tbsp pure sugar cane

Pinch of salt

Directions:

Add water and rice into the inner pot of Pressure Pot duo crisp and stir well.

Seal the pot with a pressure-cooking lid and cook on high for 3 minutes.

Once done, allow to release pressure naturally. Remove lid.

Meanwhile, heat coconut milk, sugar, and salt into the saucepan over medium heat until the sugar is dissolved. Set aside.

Add the half coconut milk mixture into the rice and stir it well.

Seal the pot with a pressure-cooking lid and cook on high for 5 minutes.

Once done, release pressure using a quick release.

Remove lid.

Serve and enjoy.

Nutrition:

Calories 299, Fat 26.7g, Carbohydrates 16.3g, Sugar 8.3g, Protein 2.8g, Cholesterol 0mg.

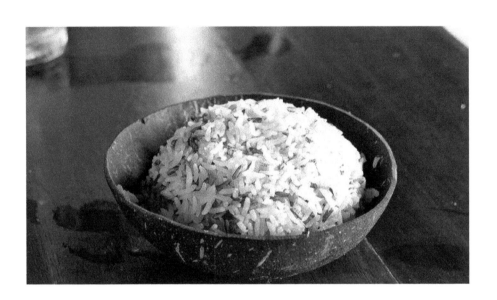

Buckwheat Cobbler

Preparation Time: 10 minutes | Cooking Time: 12 minutes | Servings: 6

Ingredients:

1/2 cup dry buckwheat

2 1/2 lbs apples, cut into chunks

1/4 tsp nutmeg

1/4 tsp ground ginger

1 1/2 tsp cinnamon

1 1/2 cups water

1/4 cup dates, chopped

Directions:

Add all ingredients into the inner pot Pressure Pot duo crisp and stir well.

Seal the pot with a pressure-cooking lid and cook on high for 12 minutes.

Once done, release pressure using a quick release. Remove lid.

Stir well and serve.

Nutrition:

Calories 119, Fat 0.6g, Carbohydrates 29.2g, Sugar 14.4g, Protein 2.1g, Cholesterol 0mg.

Perfect Strawberry Souffle

Preparation Time: 10 minutes | Cooking Time: 15 minutes | Servings: 4

Ingredients:

3 egg whites

1/2 tsp vanilla

1 tbsp sugar

2 cups strawberries

Directions:

Spray four ramekins with cooking spray and set them aside.

Add strawberries, vanilla, and sugar into the blender and blend until smooth.

In a large bowl, beat egg whites until medium peaks form. Add strawberry mixture and fold well.

Pour batter into the prepared ramekins.

Place the dehydrating tray in a multi-level air fryer basket and place basket in the Pressure Pot.

Place ramekins on a dehydrating tray.

Seal pot with air fryer lid and select bake mode then set the temperature to 350° F and timer for 15 minutes.

Serve and enjoy.

Nutrition:

Calories 49, Fat 0.3g, Carbohydrates 8.8g, Sugar 6.8g, Protein 3.2g, Cholesterol 0mg.

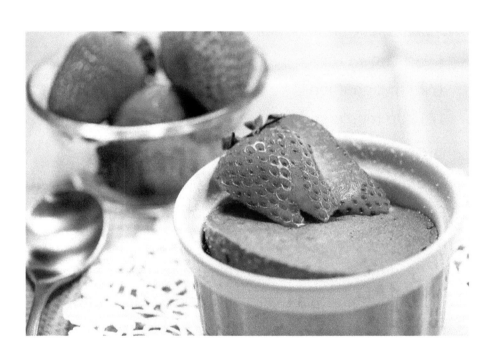

Apple Pear Crisp

Preparation time: 10 minutes | Cooking Time: 20 minutes | Servings: 4

Ingredients:

4 apples, peel, and cut into chunks

1 cup steel-cut oats

2 pears, cut into chunks

1 1/2 cup water

1/2 tsp cinnamon

1/4 cup maple syrup

Directions:

Add all ingredients into the Pressure Pot and stir well.

Seal pot with lid and cook on manual high for 10 minutes.

Once done then allow to release pressure naturally for 10 minutes then release using the quick-release method. Open the lid.

Serve warm and enjoy.

Nutrition:

Calories 306, Fat 1.9g, Carbohydrates 74g, Sugar 45.3g, Protein 3.7g, Cholesterol 0mg.

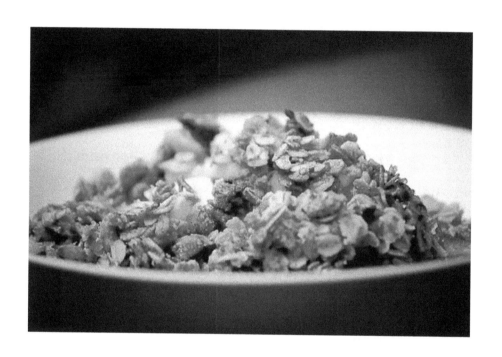

Vanilla Peanut Butter Fudge

Preparation time: 10 minutes | Cooking Time: 90 minutes | Servings: 12

Ingredients:

1 cup of chocolate chips

8.5 oz cream cheese

1/4 cup peanut butter

1/2 tsp vanilla

1/4 cup swerve

Directions:

Add all **Ingredients:** into the Pressure Pot and stir well. Seal pot with lid and cook on slow cook mode for 60 minutes.

Once done then release pressure using the quick-release method then open the lid.

Stir until smooth and cook for 30 minutes more on sauté mode.

Pour mixture into the baking pan and place in the fridge until set.

Slice and serve.

Nutrition:

Calories 177, Fat 13.9g, Carbohydrates 14.9g, Sugar 12.8g, Protein 3.9g, Cholesterol 25mg.

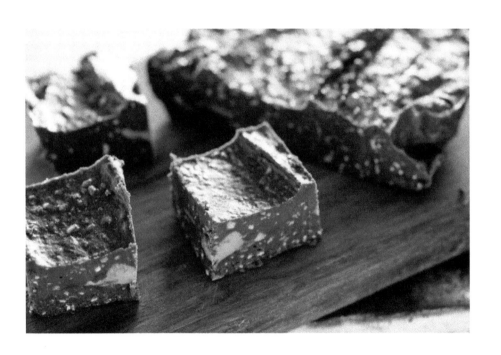